Essential Oils

A guide to aromatherapy and essential oils

Lauren Lingard

Table of Contents

Introduction 1

Chapter 1: The Must-Have List of Essential Oils 6

Chapter 2: What is Aromatherapy? 24

Chapter 3: Creative Uses of Essential Oils 37

Chapter 4: Using Essential Oils Safely 61

Chapter 5: Using Essential Oils Safely Around Your Pets 70

Conclusion 75

Introduction

You may be new to the application of essential oils, but the oils themselves are far from a new concept. Essential oils have been intertwined with our history since before even Biblical times. Many ancient cultures practiced the extraction of a plant's oils to use as our first treatment of illness as well as to address other spiritual and physical needs.

Ancient people were masters of this knowledge and had a greater understanding of the applications of essential oils than we seem to have even today. Their writings tell us that the initial uses of essential oils included medicinal, aromatic, therapeutic, and spiritual support for many cultures of people.

According to The Essential Oils Academy, the earliest use of essential oils takes place during the years 3000 to 2500 B.C. While it's true that the ancient Egyptians used many oils for embalming, culinary, beauty, and spiritual uses, there is also evidence that China and India were using essential oils at approximately the same time. Knowing that the Egyptians were so obsessed with beauty it isn't hard to believe that Cleopatra, their legendary and beautiful queen, would have used essential oils to enhance her spa treatments. Priests and ruling families in ancient Egypt wore expensive aromatics, and several of their ancient temple walls tell the tale of extracting these oils from various plants to use for many applications. Were you aware that part of the treasure found in King Tutankhamen's tomb included fifty alabaster jars that were custom-carved for essential oils? These jars must have had great value indeed, because tomb raiders took the oils and left the gold buried with the king.

Here are a few more examples of ancient cultures and their usages of essential oils:

- Roman culture has always been influenced by Greek traditions, and their use of essential oils for aromatics and health was rivaled by no other. They took several baths filled with the most exotic essential oils daily, and also indulged in massages which incorporated essential oils.

- China is known for its traditional Chinese medicine, and their usage of essential oils has been dated to around 2700 B.C. in the oldest surviving medical text penned by Shannong, the father of Chinese herbal medicine. Even today the largest producer of essential oils is China.

- During the Middle Ages the Catholic Church denounced the use of essential oils as witchcraft, forcing the monks of that era to keep their secrets of plant medicine alive in the safety of the shadows.

- After the Middle Ages (roughly 1600 to 1800), essential oils experienced a resurgence in popularity, and in Germany, France, and England they were prescribed for a variety of illnesses. The Essential Oils Academy has remarked that the first recorded lab tests regarding the antibacterial properties of essential oils took place in 1887. This test was performed because tuberculosis was running rampant in that year, but workers who processed flowers and herbs seemed to remain free of the disease, lending to the belief that oils and essences from the plants were protecting them.

- The Bible refers often to many aromatic plants; two of the most popular oils, frankincense, and myrrh, were said to be delivered as gifts after the birth of Christ. Many of our modern uses of essential oils can be traced back to these historical records.

- Fast-forward to the year 1910 in which there was a historical event in the world of essential oils: A French cosmetic chemist by the name of Rene-Maurice Gattefosse was severely injured during a lab explosion, creating gas gangrene within his tissue. He immersed his burns in a large container of lavender oil and, according to the records, that one rinse stopped the deterioration of his tissue. Because of this incident, a man who previously had no interest in essential oils and their natural healing abilities turned his attention toward their study and the effects they had while treating World War I soldiers recovering in military hospitals.

- Other French doctors, namely Jean Valnet, Pierre Franchomme, and Daniel Pénoël, were all instrumental in the continued study and use of essential oils. Valnet used essential oils to fight infection during wartime, and Franchomme along with Pénoël spent time investigating and cataloging two hundred and seventy essential oils and their medicinal properties. Their work reinvigorated interest in the practice of aromatherapy, and their book became the primary reference book for all those researching the medical benefits of essential oils.

- Doctors today in England, France, and Germany will commonly offer their patients a choice of prescription medicines, natural essential oils, or a combination of both when treating their health conditions.

Essential oils have historically proven to be man's first line of defense in medicine and have stood the test of time. Their reintroduction has inspired new clinical studies and provided us with even greater benefits. The practice of aromatherapy is quickly becoming a powerful go-to for many health care professionals.

What Can Essential Oils Be Used For?

The sky's the limit! And with new research being done all the time, there are always new applications to add. Essential oils are far more versatile than you might have ever imagined.

Essential oils are pleasantly fragrant, naturally sourced, and can affect anything in your life from the length of your lifespan right down to aiding your emotional state.

How it Works

When you inhale a fragrance, the molecules of that oil enter your nose via the air and are then absorbed by the olfactory membranes inside your nose. When your olfactory membranes become stimulated by the oil's odor molecules, it sends electrical impulses to the olfactory center located in your brain. In turn, these impulses are sent to the gustatory center, the amygdala, and the other limbic systems found within your brain.

Your limbic system is connected to many other parts of your brain, and essential oils can have a profound influence on both the physiological and psychological. A few examples of systems and symptoms which can be improved by the utilization of the essential oils include:

- Blood pressure
- Stress levels
- Hormone imbalances
- Breathing problems
- Heart rate

Chapter 1: The Must-Have List of Essential Oils

Everyone has to begin somewhere on their journey with essential oils, but where to start? There are so many to choose from that researching and selecting your first few can be a daunting experience. In truth, there's a lot to consider when choosing your oils: In some cases, it may even depend a bit on the application you wish to use it for. But this guide is designed to help narrow your options down and provide some guidance for beginners and experts alike.

Truthfully, you don't need a lot of oils when you are first getting started. By beginning with just a few of the most important essential oils, you can avoid becoming overwhelmed both financially and olfactorily.

Before we get into the must-have list, however, I want to take a moment to advise you on how to pick your oils and oil manufacturers. An oil that's cheaper may seem like a great way to save a few dollars, but be warned that you should always purchase 100% pure oil. There are brands out there that pollute the essential oil with harmful additives that will not work the way you want it to and could even end up hurting you. Unfortunately, not all essential oils are created equally.

Always read the labels thoroughly, because fake essential oils can be easy to create in a lab without a plant in sight. You may see some chemicals listed in the ingredients or even propyl glycol. These stretch the plant essences so that companies can make a substantial profit from just a small bit of oil, but the result is that the customer is using an oil that may be unhealthy and grossly manipulated.

Here are a few tips to help you discern the real from the fake essential oils:

1. **Bottle color.** Real oils are always stored in a dark-colored amber (or sometimes cobalt blue) bottle. If what you are holding in your hand is in a clear or other colored bottle, it is probably a fake.

2. **Bottle composition.** Real oils need to be stored in a glass container for two very important reasons. Firstly, real oils will melt a plastic bottle and cause a huge mess by leaking everywhere. Secondly, a bottle made of anything but glass, will leach properties into the oil which will make it impure. It should be noted that a plastic lid is fine when specifically crafted from essential oil-safe materials. Your oils are not sitting up against this lid when stored, so potential messes are avoided.

3. **Orifice reducer.** This is the contraption that is inserted at the opening of the bottle. It plays an important role because the last thing you want to do is spill the entire contents on something or pour too much of the expensive liquid accidentally. The orifice reducer will only let you access and count one drop at a time; it also protects oils from too much contact with the air which can cause oxidation. Anything without a reducer is probably a fake oil.

4. **Real essential oils come from highly recommended farms or are wild-crafted.** The quality of the oil comes from the practices followed by the farm. They should never use pesticides or toxic chemicals. The use of these can affect the purity greatly.

5. **Cost.** If you see an inexpensive price point, you can bet the oil is fake. The truth is that pure essential oils cost more because they are pure and not polluted by chemicals. Follow the adage that if it seems too good to be true, then it probably is.

6. **The smell.** Within the same brand of essential oil (for example, peppermint), you might notice that your second bottle smells stronger or weaker than your first. This is a telltale sign of good-quality products because plant quality can never be controlled while out in the field. If you find one batch smelling exactly the same as the next consistently, then it's probably created in a lab and likely to be fake. Lab-grown essential oils will smell the same every time.

7. **A Latin description.** Your essential oil label should, in addition to its name, provide the Latin designation for the plant it is derived from. So, if you have a bottle of Lavender in your hand, then it should also say Lavandula angustifolia somewhere. If the Latin is missing, the oil is most likely fake.

Always do your research and learn a bit about the company you are buying from. I spent about a year analyzing the farms and companies which create true and quality essential oils before getting into my own practice, and while I encourage you to do the same, this guide will help to expedite that process. Always check with your doctor if you are pregnant or under a doctor's care before adding essential oils into your daily routine.

The Best Essential Oils for Beginners

There are close to a hundred essential oils available for purchase today, but you will not need anywhere near that to get started. The majority of people do quite well when they stick to a shortlist of some of the most popular oils. Start with five of the most popular essential oils and build your knowledge of them. Everyone's needs are different, so top choices will vary from person to person.

Lavender (Lavandula angustifolia)

If there is a number one choice for your essential oils kit, it has got to be lavender! This plant originates in France, Utah, and Idaho, and has so many different uses that I just don't see how anyone can get along without it. Lavender is extracted by steam distillation from the flowering top of the plant. Your single bottle of lavender oil (say, fifteen milliliters) takes twenty-five square feet of lavender plants to produce!

Lavender is a soft fragrance that exudes a calm and relaxing scent, and according to a test run in 2001 by Osaka Kyoiku University, this essential oil reduces mental stress and depression. It's no surprise that lavender is the most-used essential oil in the world today. Aromatherapy promotes the use of lavender for antibacterial and antimicrobial benefits. In addition to this, lavender has medicinal properties that support antifungal, antiseptic, and anti-inflammatory applications to reduce bacteria.

This universal oil may also help arthritis, asthma, bronchitis, high blood pressure, and respiratory infections. Many people diffuse lavender every night to help with insomnia!

Peppermint (Mentha piperita)

If I had to pick my top five oils, peppermint would be my second choice. The peppermint plant originates in North America, Great Britain, and the Mediterranean area. Peppermint is extracted by steam distillation from its stems and leaves.

Peppermint oil is extremely versatile and can be used aromatically, internally, and topically. According to certified doctor of natural medicine Dr. Josh Axe, peppermint has been proven to provide antimicrobial, antioxidant, and antiviral properties. In addition, peppermint may help with the reduction of both pain and bruising. Every time you have a sore muscle or bruise from a workout or a clumsy moment, you can reach for your peppermint bottle!

The use of peppermint oil has been documented since 1,000 B.C. and today is often used for anti-nausea benefits as well as for soothing irritations in the colon and gastric lining. Many athletes find that when applied topically on their muscles, peppermint brings a cooling effect that relieves the achiness of sore muscles.

Peppermint has been used for topical pain relief and has assisted some that are troubled by fibromyalgia and myofascial pain.

Peppermint also helps clear congestion, sinusitis, asthma, colds, flus, and other respiratory ailments. Because of its respiratory benefits, peppermint oil is highly effective for seasonal allergy relief.

Other uses for peppermint oil include curbing the appetite and preventing viral infections, headaches, and skin conditions.

Since it is a strong essential oil, you should avoid contact with mucus membranes, fresh wounds, eyes, or burns.

Lemon (Citrus limon)

Citrus plants give us some of the best essential oils in existence, and they treat a wide variety of health conditions. Lemon oil is one of the most popular in the citrus essential oil family. This oil is very versatile and provides powerful antioxidant properties.

This plant originates in California and Italy, and the preferred extraction method consists of cold-pressing from the rind only. Fun fact: It takes three *thousand* lemons to produce a kilo of oil!

If a person needs to cleanse toxins from their body, lemon essential oil can be used to purify toxins and fight bacteria. Aside from the health benefits, you can drop a little in your laundry load or household cleaner for a refreshing clean smell throughout your house.

One benefit of lemon is the relief of nausea in conjunction with morning sickness. In addition, lemon can help soothe digestive problems, nourish your skin, and purify the body. If you have nagging allergies then this is the essential oil for you, since it helps relieve coughs and boost the immune system all at the same time. Lemon essential oil will also stimulate lymphatic drainage, which in turn eliminates an accumulation of fluids and diminishes coughs.

Tea Tree (Melaleuca alternifolia)

This oil is well-known for its ability to treat wounds as well as for its antiseptic properties. This is one of the top antibacterial essential oils, and it comes from Australia. The oil is produced by steam distillation of the plant's leaves. While this is a powerful antiseptic oil, you should be aware that this particular oil is a huge no-no if you own cats or dogs because it is highly toxic to them. The reason I am mentioning this now (and in more depth in chapter 5) is that many home cleaning products and cosmetic products such as shampoos, conditioners, and laundry detergents are beginning to incorporate this oil into their list of ingredients. If you have household pets, you should be aware of any potential dangers this may bring and always check labels before purchase.

In pet-free environments, tea tree oil can be topically applied to heal skin infections, and it is commonly used to kill germs, fight infections, and soothe skin conditions like eczema and psoriasis. If you have sensitive skin, keep in mind that you may experience a reaction, and you can reduce the potency of the essential oil by diluting it in a one-to-one ratio with coconut oil, canola oil, or any other carrier oil (which will be explained in depth later).

The antifungal properties of this oil lend it the ability to fight afflictions such as athlete's foot, toenail fungus, and ringworm. If you are experiencing stinky shoes, a few drops inside can help to diminish the smell. There are also reports of this oil treating or removing warts by simply applying a few drops directly on the area once or twice a day for thirty days. Should you wish to put an end to foot odor, combine a half teaspoon of coconut oil with two to three drops of tea tree oil and massage this into your feet.

Tea tree oil also is effective in getting rid of head lice!

If you have no pets, you can diffuse tea tree oil in your home. Tea tree oil should never be taken orally for any reason, as it can be poisonous if swallowed.

Orange (Citrus sinensis)

Up until now your exposure to orange oil has probably been limited to the peeling of the orange fruit. Without realizing it, you have probably smelled traces of orange oil in many of your household cleaners and cosmetic products. The plant originates in the United States, South Africa, Italy, and China, and the extraction process is centered around cold pressing the rind.

Orange oil has immune-boosting properties and is also used in many of your personal products including shampoos, lotions, and mouthwashes. Top benefits of this oil include its abilities to enhance immunity and fight cancer. All citrus-based essential oils can improve the safety of foods, even preventing the growth of E. coli bacteria.

This oil is often used as a natural remedy for high blood pressure, hypertension, and poor circulation. In addition, orange oil can help your body recover from inflammatory swelling and can be used for bone and joint pain.

If you are in need of establishing a more positive mood, increasing your pain tolerance, or if you are experiencing swelling or sore muscles, reach for your bottle of orange essential oil.

Aromatherapists have used orange oil for many years as a mild tranquilizer and a natural antidepressant. By diffusing orange oil throughout your home, inhaling it can lift your mood and bring on relaxation. Try inhaling it right after a nighttime shower to get a good night's sleep.

Cedarwood (Cedrus atlantica or Juniperus virginiana if from the Eastern red cedar)

Ancient Egyptians used cedarwood in their embalming practices, and historically in Tibet cedarwood has been used in traditional medicine and incense. The deep tones of cedarwood help calm and purify by being diffused or applied topically.

The origin of cedarwood is Morocco and the United States, and the extraction is performed by steam distilling the plant's bark.

The oil collected from cedarwood tree bark has anti-inflammatory, antifungal, and insecticidal benefits. Cedarwood is very versatile and can be useful for several different applications including hair loss, infections, and the relief of stress. It even repels moths!

If you are looking for an essential oil to add to your medical kit, cedarwood is a great choice. Between its antiseptic properties and the ability to provide arthritis relief, cedarwood can also relieve coughs, aid in the fight against acne, and help those with ADHD to focus more effectively. Cedarwood fragrance will stimulate the limbic region of the brain which affects the pineal gland, which can also create melatonin to assist in easy sleep.

Because of its woody tones, cedarwood is a very popular ingredient in many commercial perfumes. You should only use cedarwood externally since it is not a safe oil to ingest; it can cause severe issues within the digestive system.

Remember to always talk to your doctor before using any oil, especially if pregnant or nursing.

Frankincense (Boswellia carteri)

This is one of the pricier oils, but it is well worth the bang for your buck, and I would highly recommend this in any essential oil starter kit. It was among the three gifts brought by the kings for baby Jesus, and at one time this oil was more valuable than gold! In ancient days, this oil was thought to cure any ailment known to man.

The plant originates in Somalia and Yemen and is extracted by steam distillation from the gum and resin of the plant.

Medicinal properties of frankincense include being an immunity stimulant, antidepressant, and antitumoral. Among its many applications, frankincense is used to fight depression, cancer, respiratory infections, and to stimulate the immune system.

If you have never smelled frankincense before, it might remind you of a combination of pine, wood, and lemon scents. You can use frankincense oil by inhaling the oil or absorbing it through the skin (usually by mixing it with a carrier oil). In the case of this oil, a little goes a long way; know, however, that it is toxic and should never be ingested.

Frankincense is often used to reduce stress and negative emotions such as depression and anxiety. The best thing about using an oil like this is that there are no negative side effects like drowsiness or mind fog.

According to Dr. Josh Axe, a 2012 study found a natural chemical compound in frankincense named AKBA which proved to be successful in the destruction of cancer cells which had become resistant to chemotherapy.

In addition to cancer-fighting agents, frankincense can also help to prevent signs of aging and improve memory. Since it aids in lowering your body temperature and provides a calming scent, frankincense can also help you fall asleep more easily.

While there are no known side effects associated with the external use of frankincense, you should always follow any essential oil safety protocols. However, if you have blood clotting issues you should not use frankincense since it is known to have blood-thinning effects. Should you be taking anticoagulant medications, frankincense may have a negative reaction when added to your medication regimen.

Eucalyptus Globulus (Eucalyptus globulus)

There are over five hundred species of eucalyptus trees, but for this list I have chosen to include just this one. Eucalyptus trees are native to Australia and other nearby islands, and the other origin for this plant is China.

This oil is known to be a powerful antimicrobial agent, and for thousands of years the indigenous Aboriginal Australian people have used these leaves to disinfect and cover wounds. Interestingly, eucalyptus trees were planted across many parts of

Northern Africa to help stop the spread of malaria. The best extraction method for this oil is cold extraction using CO_2.

Traditional medicine was known to use eucalyptus oil to help relieve pain while acting as an analgesic agent. In addition, it has been used to reduce inflammation and improve respiratory conditions.

Thanks to these benefits and its fresh, natural scent, eucalyptus oil is prevalent in many commercial products including healing ointments, vapor rubs, perfumes, and cleaning products.

If you are plagued by respiratory conditions, then you will enjoy the oil's effectiveness against COPD, asthma, bronchitis, sinusitis, and the common cold or flu. Because eucalyptus oil helps to stimulate your immune system you may find that using it makes it much easier to breathe when your nose is congested. By diffusing the oil, eucalyptus can help you to sleep when you are struggling to breathe through a blocked nose.

Do you have seasonal allergies? This oil is often used to alleviate those symptoms, including headaches and muscle pain. It can also be used to soothe insect bites.

You can add drops of eucalyptus while cleaning your house, too. Since it has antimicrobial properties it can provide protection against bacteria, viruses, and fungi. Hopefully you never experience a rat infestation, but just in case you do, eucalyptus oil can fix that. Just add twenty drops of eucalyptus oil to a spray bottle filled with plain water and apply it to areas that might attract rats. Do take care if you have cats, though; eucalyptus can be irritating to them, too.

If you have sensitive skin, you should utilize the practice of diluting eucalyptus oil with a carrier oil before applying it to your skin. Because the facial area can be especially sensitive, you should avoid using it on any facial area in its pure form. You can also diffuse it, but like many other essential oils, it is not safe for internal use.

Geranium (Pelargonium graveolens)

This essential oil was used by ancient Egyptians to produce beautiful skin, alleviate anxiety, and heal skin conditions. It is a sweet-smelling oil that can affect you by lifting troublesome moods, lessening your fatigue, and lending you emotional wellness.

The origin of this plant is Egypt and India, and the extraction method is steam distillation from the flowers and leaves of the plant.

Its medicinal properties include being an antioxidant, anti-inflammatory, and antibacterial. This oil can be used topically alone, but it is recommended that you use a carrier oil and be sure to avoid the eye area if you apply it to your face.

Geranium essential oil provides stress relief, aids in alleviating depression and inflammation, improves circulation, and reduces blood pressure. There are ongoing studies demonstrating the effect of geranium oil on neuroinflammatory illnesses such as Alzheimer's. So far, the study has suggested that geranium oil might be beneficial to prevent Alzheimer's and Dementia. In other tests, scientists are studying the effects of geranium oil on shingles.

You can add a few drops of geranium oil to your shampoo, conditioner, or body soap to provide a sweet lingering smell after your shower.

Want to make geranium oil at home? All you need are a few leaves of a geranium plant (the more you use, the stronger the fragrance). Wash all the leaves completely and dry them in a clean washcloth. After the leaves have dried, use a mortar and pestle to grind the leaves until they are completely mashed and let that sit for a few hours. After that, add a carrier oil such as coconut or jojoba oil to the smashed leaves. Cover the mixture and let it sit for two weeks in a cool, dry place. The first thing you will notice is the lovely scent of your newly made oil. Finish by draining the leaves and keeping them in an air-tight glass container.

German Chamomile (Matricaria recutita)

The two types of chamomile applied in today's medicines are German chamomile and Roman chamomile (see below). German chamomile plants were originally from Egypt, Hungary, Utah, and Idaho, and the extraction method is steam distillation from the flowers of the plant.

Egyptians dedicated festivals to this plant because of its healing properties, and Germans have used chamomile for centuries to alleviate digestive issues. Almost every culture has used this medicinal herb to fight different maladies including inflammation, allergies, and general pain. If you have ever felt poorly and brewed yourself up a cup of chamomile tea, then you know that it can help with anxiety, depression, and insomnia.

Chamomile essential oil can also be used at home to soothe skin conditions and provide you with a source of antioxidants that may create better immune function. This oil can also aid in liver and gallbladder health.

This essential oil can be diffused, added to water or food, or applied topically, as this is one of the most gentle oils used in aromatherapy. You can even use it in the bathtub! Just add five drops each of chamomile and bergamot oil in the palm of your hand and rub this into your muscles. Soak in the bath for at least fifteen minutes to maximize the benefits and you will emerge with a calmed mind and soothed muscles.

Roman Chamomile (Anthemis nobilis)

This is another essential oil that I recommend beginners to seek out. Roman chamomile plants originated in France and Utah, and the oil is produced by steam distilling the flowering top.

Its medical properties include being a relaxant, an anti-inflammatory, antiparasitic, and antibacterial. You can gain benefits from this oil by diffusing it at home or applying it topically to the skin.

Its fragrance promotes a calming effect and relaxes an individual, aiding against anxiety, depression, ADHD, and insomnia. Should you find that you need to calm your nerves, Roman chamomile essential oil may be an excellent tool for you to use. By diffusing and exposing yourself to this aromatherapy treatment, you should see an improvement in sleep quality. If you suffer from insomnia, this can help you experience a more restful state by helping you to feel calm and drowsy.

In addition to its calming effects this oil may also help relieve allergies, reduce the symptoms of PMS, and relieve arthritic pains.

Roman chamomile can be applied to the skin, diffused, or taken internally and has a sweet, fresh, apple-like aroma. Since this is one of the oldest and most versatile oils, it has a long history of being used to treat a multitude of conditions.

Rosemary (Rosmarinus officinalis CT Cineole)

The rosemary plant dates as far back as 500 B.C. and originates from France, Asia, and the United States. Rosemary was used to protect people during the 15th-century plague, it has been burned as incense, and at one point it was even believed to ward off the devil.

The extraction method for rosemary oil is to use steam to distill the oil from the leaves. Rosemary is applied to relieve infectious disease, liver conditions, hepatitis, acne, Alzheimer's, and throat or lung infections.

The aroma of rosemary is woodsy, and some describe it as a combination of pine, lemon, and camphor. Although rosemary is most often identified as being used for cooking, it also has therapeutic uses that help to protect the liver. It is anti-inflammatory, antifungal, antibacterial, anticancer, and antidepressant.

Besides having a pleasant taste and fragrance, rosemary is often used to help relieve pain, inflammation, gastrointestinal pains, respiratory issues, and anxiety. Should you be taking a high blood pressure medication, it is advised that you do not use rosemary.

Rose (Rosa damascena)

Roses provide more than just a declaration of love for your significant other and a pleasant, fragrant smell. The plant originates from Bulgaria and Turkey and the distillation process from the rose petals involves two different steps. An Arab physician by the name of Avicenna (c. 980-1037 A.D.) was the first to distill rose oil and even authored a book on the healing brought about by its use.

The application of rose oil can improve general skin health, allergies, feelings of grief, and nervous tension. In addition, rose oil can be anti-inflammatory, anti-HIV, anti-aging, and an antioxidant. In the cosmetic industry, rose oil has been used to reduce scarring, wrinkles, acne, and other skin conditions.

Once you smell rose oil you will never forget the rich floral scent reminiscent of something both sweet and spicy. That's why this oil is used in so many perfumes on the market today.

Rose oil possesses mood-boosting abilities and can help with depression and anxiety. This essential oil is often used to relieve pain associated with menstrual periods or to boost a struggling libido.

You can use this essential oil either topically or aromatically, but it is not advised to use it internally.

Black Pepper (Piper nigrum)

While historically black pepper was used by ancient Egyptians for mummification, we use this oil today for other valuable pursuits. This plant originates in Madagascar, Sri Lanka, England, and India, and the essence is extracted by steam distillation from the fruit of the plant. There is a second and more preferred way to extract this oil, which is through CO_2 extraction. This second method ensures that chemicals like ethanol and hexane are left out of the processing of the oil.

The uses for this plant go far beyond a sprinkle of pepper on our morning eggs; research has pointed to possible benefits for enhancing circulation and more. The most active component of black pepper is called piperine, which has been shown to have possible anti-cancerous properties.

Black pepper is known to stimulate the metabolism, making it an excellent tool to combat obesity, but the benefits don't stop there. This essential oil is also used for arthritis, nerve and muscle pain, and fatigue.

This essential oil can be taken internally, inhaled, or applied topically. There is an added benefit for those trying to kick the cigarette habit, since black pepper oil may help smokers reduce their cravings for cigarettes as well as the anxiety caused by nicotine withdrawal. The best method to reduce nicotine cravings is to diffuse the oil or inhale directly from the bottle when the urge strikes.

You can expect it to have a warm, spicy, and musky aroma and to create a warming sensation. You can use it with a carrier oil such as coconut oil, jojoba oil, or almond oil. Should you need to increase circulation and blood flow to an area, simply add three to five drops of black pepper oil to a warm compress and apply to the injured area. This application also applies to muscle injuries and tendonitis.

Chapter 2: What is Aromatherapy?

The practice of aromatherapy is believed to have its roots in the ancient religious ceremonies of burning fragrant needles, bark, and leaves.

In addition, certain tribes learned that adding flowers and plants to their meat as it cooked over the fire added more flavor to their food. Through experimentation they found that certain plants when mixed with fat would heal their wounds more efficiently than unscented fat. This was likely the beginning of our modern scented body lotions. The wearer likely found that it changed their emotions for the better.

We have a lot to thank our ancient ancestors for. Their curiosity and experimentation in combining one thing with another ended up being the foundation for modern aromatherapy.

Aromatherapy has grown to become one of the most important cornerstones of alternative medicine, and is defined as using natural oils that are extracted from flowers, bark, stems, roots, and leaves to improve physical and psychological well-being.

Of course, research on how effective aromatherapy is has its limits, and is sometimes contested within and outside of the holistic health community. Oils will affect every individual differently, and it is up to the individual to discern the health benefits of utilizing essential oils and to experiment with different application methods to find what best fits them. It's important to understand that the holistic healing brought about by aromatherapy walks the line between art and science, and can improve both physical and mental health. Aromatherapy treatment can be applied in the following manners:

- Diffusers
- Aromatic spritzers
- Inhalers
- Bathing salts
- Body oils, creams, or lotions used for topical application or massages
- Facial steamers
- Hot and cold compresses

If you suffer from anxiety, depression, insomnia, or chronic health problems, why wouldn't you want to give aromatherapy a chance? Aromatherapy has a large offering of benefits. Provided you use essential oils responsibly, they can have a very positive impact on your health and well-being.

What is an Aromatherapist?

An aromatherapist is a person who is trained in the ability to combine aromas to lead a client toward better physical health. With their eye for detail in the art and science of combining oils, they will create a regimen for you in response to questions about your health and lifestyle. In doing so they will help you manage your symptoms by tailoring oil choices to your specific needs.

A personal aromatherapy program will be able to work in conjunction with any medical care or treatment you are already receiving. Just make sure that you talk to your doctor prior to beginning any aromatherapy sessions.

Diffusing

The best way to use essential oils is in a diffuser. Want to calm down after a hectic day at work? Fill your diffuser with water and add both lavender and peppermint oils. This combination can provide you with a nice calm feeling after a rough day.

Conversely, if you are just beginning your day and need to get yourself motivated, reach for a nice citrus smell like orange.

I feel that it is important to mention that there are different ways to diffuse, and the most effective (besides direct inhalation from the bottle and/or an ultrasonic diffuser) is using a cold-air fan diffuser.

Many people don't realize the poisons they put into their homes when using plug-in air freshener devices. Not only are these full of harmful chemicals but they can be dangerous for pets (not to mention fire hazards). I cannot for the life of me understand why people use them when there are perfectly good essential oils that smell great *and* come with health and wellness benefits!

There is a powerful neurological connection between scent and memory. Try to remember back to sitting in your mother's kitchen when you were a child. Can you recall the smell of chocolate chip cookies being baked? Can you remember the colors of the walls, the apron your mother was wearing, or the excitement of being allowed to lick the spoon? While there is no such thing as a chocolate chip essential oil, scents such as cinnamon, oregano, and basil might bring back memories such as this. Likewise, by diffusing new scents or combinations, you will be able to build new memories and positive experiences. If you grow to associate the smell of lavender with being calm, then you can use that scent-memory link to later calm yourself down from an anxious state by wafting lavender under your nose. This is yet another reason why aromatherapy and diffusing can be such an effective healing method.

Direct Inhalation

Simply open a bottle of your chosen essential oil and inhale. Waft your hand in the air above the bottle's orifice to dilute the scent if it's too powerful to inhale directly. You can also put a few drops of oil in the palm of your hands, rub them together, and then cup them gently over your nose and mouth to inhale the scent. You can even place a few drops in hot (not boiling) water and inhale the vapor produced.

Cold-Air Fan

A cold-air fan will diffuse by blowing cool air through an essential oil pad. This releases essential oil molecules into the air around you.

Ultrasonic Diffusers

This type of diffuser combines the various benefits of an air purifier, humidifier, and an aromatherapy diffuser. It works by taking a mixture of water and essential oils and dispersing them into the air. These diffusers typically have an automatic shut-off when the unit has run out of water, and you can experience your aromatherapy session while you sleep. Be sure to use distilled or purified water, since the ultrasonic vibrations will also vaporize any impurities in the water and cause them to be inhaled as well.

Aromatic Spritzer

This form of aromatherapy utilizes a combination of essential oils and water. Spritzers are an easy way to carry several oils with you, and you can use them to refresh the air in a room, reduce undesirable odors in the air, quickly soothe emotional states, and purify new locations such as hotel rooms.

A lot of us spend way too much time in our cars; instead of getting those overpowering, dangling commercial air fresheners, make a spritzer just for your car! With all the stresses of driving home after work, you might feel tired and drained; an aromatherapy spritzer can deliver some positive energy and make your commute a happier experience.

Aromatic spritzers are simple to make. Just add 5 to 8 drops of an essential oil or 3 to 4 drops of multiple essential oils per ounce of water. Add all these to an aromatherapy glass spritzer bottle which you should be able to find online or at your local health store. Shake before using.

Aromatherapy Inhalers

Thanks to the convenience of the internet, you can purchase these inhalers already pre-made, or purchase empty containers to make on your own.

These are handy because they are small in size and discreet enough to slip into your pocket. Inhaler sticks contain a wick inside that is meant to contain essential oils. This wick is contained and topped off with a cap that makes it simple to place into your nose. Place the inhaler stick into your nostril and draw in a deep breath.

Easy to Make Aromatherapy Inhalers

1. **Allergies?** To a blank wick, add one drop each of lemon, lavender, and peppermint essential oils.

2. **Need sleep?** Add a single drop of cinnamon, lemon, and grapefruit essential oils.

3. **Anxiety?** We all have those days! Try adding one drop each of lavender, ylang-ylang, and sandalwood together to ease your worries.

4. **Headaches?** Use one drop each of peppermint, rosemary, and lavender essential oils.

5. **Suffering from sinus problems?** Add one drop each of tea tree, eucalyptus, and peppermint.

Bathing Salts

There is something soothing about relaxing in a tub of bath salts brimming with essential oils. It's time to ease your stress and possibly your blood pressure while enjoying a hot soak. Fast-forward to chapter three to view a couple of my favorite recipes for making my own bath salts, but feel free to experiment and use some of your favorite oils.

Body Oils & Lotions

It's pretty easy to create homemade lotions using essential oils. The best part is that you can customize them with any scent you like. In chapter three I have included directions on making my favorite, peppermint lotion!

Facial Steamers

One way to use essential oils that is often overlooked is through facial steaming. This practice dates back to ancient Egyptian times.

Adding essential oils to your facial steamer will enhance your beauty regime. You can soften your skin and enjoy many other benefits. You can use steamers on any type of skin, but if you have sensitive skin, rosacea, or sunburned skin you should probably avoid using a steamer.

Which Essential Oils Should You Use?

- **Tea tree oil.** Used for eye and ear infections, clogged pores including whiteheads and blackheads, colds, sore throat, acne, and rashes.

- **Lemon oil.** Aides against allergies, oily skin, and skin blemishes.

- **Lavender oil.** Soothes and beautifies your skin.

- **Peppermint oil.** Effective in easing migraines, sore throats, difficulties breathing, allergies, clogged noses and sinuses, colds, coughs, and flus.

- **Eucalyptus oil.** Able to combat all the same things listed above for peppermint.

- **Geranium oil.** Used as a skin beautifier, aids in the treatment of hormonal and cystic acne, and clears clogged pores.

- **Patchouli oil.** This oil will bring calmness to your body.

- **Orange oil.** May be effective in calming an upset stomach.

If you want to be more updated than the old mixing bowl, there are plenty of facial steamers on the market and they can be found online and at many of your local retailers.

Keep in mind that you can also use combinations! Lavender and Roman chamomile is an excellent combination to use just before bedtime. Both oils provide calming effects and will help you fall asleep easier.

Targeting Skin Types

Below, I have added some information on the various skin types and oils that work best with them.

Dry Skin

Some people naturally have dry skin, and it can be seasonal or depend upon the climate. Top essential oils for dry skin include sandalwood and frankincense. Lavender will provide moisturizing and anti-inflammatory properties that will help your skin repair itself through hydration. Finally, German chamomile contains chamazulene, which decreases inflammation and increases moisture.

Oily Skin

Oily skin is irritating, and nobody likes dealing with it. The good news is that there are oils to use that will make it easier to manage. Things that exacerbate oily skin include humidity, heat, and hormones. It may seem odd to contemplate using oils to make your skin less oily, but these will help! Rosemary possesses vital ingredients that help prevent excess oils from being produced. In addition, the use of clary sage is another popular oil for combating and controlling oil overproduction.

Sensitive Skin

If you suffer from sensitive skin, you should always use oils that provide nourishing and restorative properties. The best oils to work with sensitive skin are sandalwood and frankincense. Sandalwood has excellent anti-inflammatory properties and can provide moisture; this is why it's a popular ingredient in face washes and shaving creams. Frankincense is healing and will work to manage skin issues to provide a more even complexion.

Example of an Essential Oil Facial Steam

<u>Ingredients:</u>

- 4 cups of boiling water
- 2 drops of lavender oil
- 2 drops of tea tree oil

<u>Directions:</u>

1. Wash your face before a face steam.

2. Add the boiling water to a large heatproof bowl on a table in a comfortable place where you can sit and relax.

3. Add essential oils to the water just before you are ready to experience the session as they will begin to evaporate as soon as they touch the water.

4. Create a tent over your head, shoulders, and the bowl using a bath towel. You should keep your face about 12 to 18 inches from the bowl in order to prevent getting burned from the rising steam. If you get too close to the contents,

it can lead to increased blood flow and broken capillaries. Use caution!

5. It's time to relax. Close your eyes and take a deep breath. Enjoy the benefits for 5 to 10 minutes or until the water cools.

<u>Optional Blends:</u>

You can change the oils in the above facial steam for different benefits.

- Use two drops each of eucalyptus and lavender for breathing benefits.
- Use two drops each of lemon and geranium to clear your skin.
- Use two drops each of frankincense and Roman chamomile to calm your body.

Added Benefits from a Face Steam

- **Added circulation.** Hot steam will dilate blood vessels providing strong blood and oxygen flow through your circulatory system.

- **Releases acne-causing bacteria.** Skin will attract dirt, grime, and bacteria, causing pores to clog and acne to form. Because steaming helps unclog pores, it will reduce how often and how severely you develop acne.

- **Releases sinus congestion.** If you are sick, face steams will provide relief from the symptoms of a cough or cold.

- **Provides cleansing.** Naturally, steaming will cause your body to sweat, which will open up your pores, purge toxins, and give your skin a healthy glow.

- **It's soothing.** There is nothing better than taking a few moments to experience some relaxing downtime. Add lavender to add a sense of calm and serenity to your steam.

Hot & Cold Compresses

Compresses are a basic treatment that consists of folding a piece of material such as a washcloth or small towel into a makeshift pad and wetting it with hot or cold water depending upon the treatment desired. These will help with muscular pain, increasing circulation, relieving a buildup of fluid, and reducing pain from things like sprains.

Hot Compresses

Generally, these are used for treating muscle pain, old injuries, menstrual cramps, and toothaches. Use hot water, as warm as you can stand but being careful not to burn yourself, then add four drops of your chosen essential oil. Use your folded material and place it on top of the water, allowing it to soak it up. Wring out the excess water and place the compress over the area to be treated.

You can cover the compress with cling wrap or another towel to help keep it in place. If you are trying to treat something in an awkward place you may want to lightly wrap it with a bandage to keep it on the desired spot.

Cold Compresses

These are used for recent injuries like sprains, bruising, swelling, and headaches. Cold compresses are made in the same manner as hot compresses, using ice or refrigerated water in place of hot water. Replace the application when it has heated up to your body's temperature. If using ice, you can apply your essential oil with a carrier and then proceed to ice.

My typical oils to use when I am treating an injury are peppermint and lavender, but depending upon what you are trying to accomplish, you have plenty of essential oils to choose from.

Chapter 3: Creative Uses of Essential Oils

In the last chapter I talked about aromatherapy and diffusing, but there are more ways to use essential oils than just inhaling them. Aromatherapy's benefits are not limited to the powerful scent-memory neurological link. Here are some other creative ways you can use essential oils:

- Got tag residue? Scrub away that sticky stuff! Apply a couple of drops of lemon essential oil and wipe away any leftovers.

- Shine up dry hair. Who doesn't want their hair to look great? Place a few drops of cedarwood essential oil in your hand, rub your palms together to warm it up, and massage it into your scalp for healthier hair.

- Use some essential oil blends in the tub! (See below)

- Spice up your home cleaning. Any citrus oil is fantastic to add to your cleaning regime, especially lemon or orange essential oils. You should not use essential oils on granite or stone as many of them could damage these surfaces.

- Is your evening moisturizer missing something? Add a drop of rose essential oil to your nightly routine to give you healthier-looking skin.

- Diffuse! If you are in need of a good night's rest, place some oils such as lavender, cedarwood, German chamomile, or vetiver in your diffuser for a peaceful sleep. If your dog or cat sleeps in your room, you should double check that whatever oil you use will not harm your furry friends.

- Bring more flavor to the kitchen. You can add a small amount of oregano essential oil to your favorite Italian dish. Many people don't realize that you can use many of your essential oils in your favorite recipes! Just make sure you double-check that all oils you add to food are safe for internal use.

- Make personalized essential oil roll-ons. This is a perfect way to take your essential oils with you daily. Begin by buying empty roller bottles (the first place that comes to mind is Amazon, but your health store may be able to give you a lead on where to find them locally). Add ten to fifteen drops of your chosen essential oil and then fill the rest of your bottle with the carrier oil of your choice.

- Make your own skincare products.

- Make your own cleaning products.

- Create an essential oil spray to use as a quick air freshener.

Helpful Recipes

I have gathered together some recipes using essential oils that incorporate household cleaners, shower gels, soaps, and lotions. Enjoy!

Bruise Cream with Arnica & Bilberry

If you've never had a bruise, then you just aren't human. When you inevitably get a bruise, you can always reach for your essential oils!

<u>Ingredients:</u>

- ⅓ cup jojoba oil
- ¼ cup arnica oil
- ¼ cup shea butter
- ⅛ cup coconut oil
- 3 to 4 drops comfrey oil
- 1 500 milligram bromelain capsule
- 1 tsp bilberry extract
- 10 drops frankincense essential oil
- ⅛ to ¼ cup purified water (depending on desired consistency)

Directions:

1. To a double boiler add jojoba oil and shea butter. As the mixture softens, use a wire whisk to blend well.

2. Transfer the mixture to a small mixing bowl, add the arnica oil, and blend.

3. Add the coconut oil and blend.

4. Add the comfrey oil and blend.

5. Break open the bromelain capsule and add the contents to the mixture. Stir.

6. Add the bilberry extract and the frankincense essential oils. Blend well.

7. After all the ingredients are blended, slowly add the water a little at a time, continuing to blend well.

8. Adjust the amount of water you add to get your desired consistency.

9. Transfer the mixture into a glass jar and keep the container in your refrigerator. This helps to keep the mixture consistent. When you want to use it, just set it out for a few minutes before use, allowing it to soften.

Detox in Your Tub!

Ever fantasize about sitting in a bubble bath after a long hard day? Just substitute those bubbles for some essential oils and your positive results will be assured. There is no need to go to a high-priced spa when you can achieve all those benefits right in your own bathtub.

Essential oils can rid your body of impurities through raindrop techniques (described in chapter five), and this effect can also be achieved by soaking in an oil-infused bath. If you have about forty minutes to allow the oils to work their magic, you will love the results. Why forty minutes? It will take your body around twenty minutes to rid itself of all the toxins that have built up in your system, and the last twenty will allow you to absorb all the benefits found in your water. You will emerge feeling like a whole new person.

Want to create a luxurious experience for a friend? These can make for some fantastic gifts! If you are giving these as gifts, make sure they are labeled appropriately with instructions for use, the amount to be used per bath, and all health and safety warnings associated with the oils contained within.

Eucalyptus & Vanilla Bath Salts

This smells great and can double as an anti-inflammatory and decongestant. *Tip: Take care to get up slowly, as sometimes Epsom salts can make you feel a bit lightheaded if you are not used to soaking in them.*

Ingredients:

- 1 cup Epsom salt
- ½ cup baking soda
- 3 drops eucalyptus oil
- 8 drops vanilla in jojoba oil

Directions:

1. Add all ingredients together in a large sealable plastic bag.

2. Seal or pinch the top of the bag closed and massage the contents until well mixed.

3. Transfer from the plastic bag to a glass container with a lid.

4. Use one spoonful for each bath.

Lemon & Rosemary

This is refreshing to use during the summer months and will help the user to relax. *Tip: Take care to get up slowly, as sometimes Epsom salts can make you feel a bit lightheaded if you are not used to soaking in them.*

Ingredients:

- 2 cups Epsom salt
- ½ cup baking soda
- 2 to 3 tsp rosemary, fresh and finely chopped
- 6 to 8 drops lemon essential oil

- 2 - 3 tbsp lemon zest (optional)

Directions:

1. Combine Epsom salt, baking soda, and half of the lemon oil drops. Mix well.

2. Add the additional drops, the chopped rosemary, and the lemon zest and mix again.

3. Store in a glass airtight container.

4. Use a spoonful for each bath.

Lavender & Eucalyptus Bath Blend

This is a perfect blend for a cold day when you are fighting a cold or flu. Even if you are just experiencing a stressful day, this can help ease your worries. *Tip: Take care to get up slowly, as sometimes Epsom salts can make you feel a bit lightheaded if you are not used to soaking in them.*

Ingredients:

- 2 cups Epsom salts
- ½ cup lavender, dried
- 5 to 6 drops lavender oil
- 10 drops eucalyptus oil

Directions:

1. Combine all ingredients in a bowl.

2. Store in a glass airtight container.

3. Add a spoonful or more as needed to a full bathtub with very warm water.

4. Soak for at least 20 to 30 minutes.

Create Your Own Shower Gel

For those of you that don't soak in a tub, here is a recipe for a shower gel to spice up your morning or evening routine!

Orange Shower Gel with Shea Butter

Ingredients:

- 2 tbsp shea butter
- 2 tbsp jojoba oil or almond oil
- 1 tsp coconut oil
- ¼ cup Castile soap
- 1 tbsp vegetable glycerin
- 1 tsp xanthan gum
- ¼ cup warm distilled water
- 12 drops orange essential oil

Directions:

1. In a small pan add the shea butter and melt on low heat.

2. Add jojoba oil, almond oil, and coconut oil. Mix well and then pour the mixture into a medium-sized bowl. Sprinkle the xanthan gum (a thickening agent) into the bowl. Allow this to sit for around a minute.

3. Place all the contents into an immersion blender. Pulse for one or two minutes to dissolve the gum into the butter and oil mixture.

4. Add the Castile soap (a natural vegetable-based soap), vegetable glycerin, and warm water. Blend for about two minutes. What you should see is a creamy-looking lotion.

5. For the last step, add the orange essential oil. This will add a wonderful citrus smell to your shower gel.

6. Pour the shower gel mix into a soap dispenser. Since the ingredients may separate a little after sitting, you may want to shake it before you use it. Because your mixture contains no preservatives you should use it within a few weeks, but you will emerge from your showers invigorated and ready to roll.

When You Just Love Peppermint!

Peppermint oil can stimulate circulation to your skin, balance oily skin, and makes you feel refreshed which is why it's a great choice to use in your cosmetics.

Peppermint oil is found in many of our lotions, foot baths, and herbal soaps for a very good reason. It helps improve concentration, soothe tired muscles, and reduce mental fatigue. Here are a few of my favorite peppermint recipes!

Peppermint Soap

Ingredients:

- 2 lbs. of a glycerin soap base
- 1 tbsp peppermint leaves, dried
- ½ tsp peppermint oil
- Red liquid soap coloring or a few shavings of red solid soap coloring

Directions:

1. Cut the glycerin soap into 1-inch squares and place them in a double boiler over low heat to melt.

2. Stir constantly until melted, but do not allow the soap to simmer or boil.

3. Remove from the heat and add the dried peppermint leaves, peppermint essential oil, and soap coloring.

4. Stir constantly while you add these ingredients, then pour the soap mixture into soap molds.

5. Set this aside for 4 to 8 hours allowing the soap to completely set.

6. Wrap your finished product in cheesecloth until you are ready to use.

Peppermint Lotion

Enjoy this soothing product by massaging a small amount of the lotion gently into the skin. Use small circular motions for best results.

Ingredients:

- 1 tsp peppermint leaves, dried
- 1 ½ cups boiling water
- ⅓ cup almond oil
- 1 ounce beeswax, grated
- 2 drops peppermint essential oil
- 1 drop red food coloring
- Glass jar with lid

Directions:

1. Place the dried peppermint leaves in the bottom of a Pyrex measuring cup, then pour the boiling water over the top of the leaves. Cover this and allow it to steep for 15 minutes before straining into another 2-ounce Pyrex cup.

2. Warm the almond oil in the top of a double boiler over low heat. Add the grated beeswax and stir the mixture until melted.

3. Remove the pan from the heat source and add 2 ounces of peppermint tea. Beat this mixture constantly with a wire whisk until it is well combined.

4. Stir in the peppermint essential oil and the food coloring until well blended.

5. Transfer the entire mixture to a glass storage jar and store in a cool, dark place.

Pamper Your Skin

With all the sun and air impurities floating around, you really need to pamper your skin. We all dream of having perfect skin, but for most of us it's a goal to strive for rather than a gift we're born with. Luckily, I have a few recipes here to help in achieving that goal.

Frankincense for Anti-Aging

Frankincense essential oil is an excellent choice to use for skin conditions. It may reduce scars, acne, redness, and skin irritation.

Ingredients:

- 1 tsp GMO-free vitamin C powder
- 1 tsp filtered water
- 1 ½ tbsp aloe vera gel
- ⅛ tsp vitamin E oil
- 5 drops frankincense essential oil

Directions:

1. Blend the vitamin C powder and filtered water in a bowl using a wire whisk.

2. Add the aloe vera gel and blend well.

3. Add the vitamin E oil and frankincense essential oil. Mix all the ingredients until well blended.

4. Use a funnel and transfer your mixture into a small cobalt or amber bottle which will reduce light exposure to the product.

Apply the mixture at night and make sure to remove it in the morning, as exposure to the sun while wearing the product could cause skin sensitivity. When you begin applications, you may want to start with a small area of skin every other night to ensure that your skin is not sensitive to the mixture. You will notice results from within just a few weeks to up to three months.

Tea Tree Oil Face Wash

Tea tree oil is known for its ability to soothe inflammatory skin conditions, sores, insect bites, and sunburn.

<u>Ingredients:</u>

- 1 tbsp coconut oil
- 3 tbsp honey
- 1 tbsp organic apple cider vinegar
- 20 drops tea tree essential oil
- 2 capsules of live probiotics

<u>Directions:</u>

1. Mix all the ingredients together with a hand blender.

2. Pour the mixture into a glass container to store. Keep it in a cool place.

All-Natural Moisturizer for Oily Skin

<u>Ingredients:</u>

- 3 ounces jojoba oil
- 1 ounce shea butter
- 1 ounce tamanu oil

- 5 drops rosemary oil
- 3 drops peppermint oil

Directions:

1. Using a double boiler, melt the shea butter over low heat.

2. Add the jojoba oil and blend until the mixture is combined.

3. Remove from the heat, then add the tamanu oil and blend it into the mixture using a fork or small spatula.

4. Add the essential oils and blend until well mixed.

5. Remove the finished product from the pan and place it in a small, lidded glass jar.

6. Store your product in a cool, dark place and it should last for a few months.

Cooking with Essential Oils

You may feel hesitant about adding essential oils to your kitchen concoctions, because what happens if you add too much? Have no fear, these are some of my favorite recipes perfected over time!

From breakfast to dessert and all the courses in between, you will be able to find a recipe or two that tingles your taste buds.

Raspberry Lemon Ricotta Pancakes

Ingredients:

- 1 ¾ cups flour
- 1 tbsp baking powder
- 3 tbsp sugar
- ¼ tsp kosher salt
- 2 large eggs
- 2 to 3 drops lemon essential oil
- 2 tbsp canola oil
- ⅔ cups ricotta cheese
- ⅔ cups whole milk
- 1 tsp vanilla extract
- 1 cup fresh raspberries

Directions:

1. Whisk together the flour, baking powder, sugar, and salt in a medium bowl. Set aside.

2. In a large bowl whisk together eggs, lemon oil, canola oil, ricotta cheese, whole milk, and vanilla extract until completely combined.

3. Stir in the dry ingredients to the wet and do not overmix. Your pancake batter should appear lumpy. Fold in the raspberries.

4. Preheat your griddle or large non-stick skillet over medium heat. While cooking, use a non-stick cooking spray and then pour ¼ cup of the batter on the cooking

surface. Do not overcrowd the surface and work in batches. Cook until bubbles form in the batter, approximately 3 to 4 minutes. Flip the pancakes and cook for about 2 to 3 additional minutes. Remove from the heated surface and transfer to a plate.

5. Top your pancakes with your choice of butter, maple syrup, fresh raspberries, or something else that you enjoy!

Vinaigrette Salad Dressing

Ingredients:

- ⅓ cup extra virgin olive oil
- ¾ cup organic apple cider vinegar
- 2 cloves garlic, minced
- ⅓ cup honey mustard
- ¼ cup honey
- 2 tsp Dijon mustard
- ½ tsp salt
- 1 tsp black pepper
- 3 drops Lemongrass essential oil
- 4 drops Dill essential oil

Directions:

1. Mix all of the above ingredients in a quart-sized jar. Shake well. Refrigerate overnight.

Roasted Chicken with Lemon & Thyme

Ingredients:

- 1 whole chicken
- 4 tbsp extra virgin olive oil
- 4 drops lemon essential oil
- 4 drops thyme essential oil
- dried oregano, to taste
- 1 lemon, sliced
- 1 onion, sliced

Directions:

1. Preheat your oven to 350°.

2. Mix the oils, salt, and pepper in a small bowl and set aside.

3. Place the chicken in a roasting pan with the breast side up. Remove anything in the cavity area.

4. With a silicone basting brush, cover the entire outside of the chicken with the oil mixture. Should there be any mix left over, pour it into the cavity of the chicken. If desired, sprinkle the chicken with a bit of dried oregano.

5. Place the slices of lemons and onions in the bottom of the roasting pan and some in the cavity of the chicken.

6. Add some water to barely cover the bottom of the pan.

7. Place the chicken in the oven and cook until the internal temperature of the bird reaches 180° (Roughly an hour and 45 minutes depending upon the size of the chicken).

8. Remove the pan from the oven and allow the chicken to rest 10 minutes before slicing.

Keto & Paleo Friendly Instant Pot Sesame Orange Chicken

When you have a taste for something from a Western Chinese restaurant, this recipe allows you to enjoy a dish that makes you feel like you are indulging in Chinese takeout without the added sodium, fat, or MSG.

Ingredients:

- 2 tbsp avocado or coconut oil
- ⅔ cup coconut aminos
- 3 tbsp tomato paste
- ¼ cup raw honey (omit for keto diet)
- 4 cloves garlic, minced
- 2 inches fresh ginger, grated and peeled
- ½ cup bone broth (or you can substitute ¾ cup orange juice)
- ½ tsp black pepper
- A pinch of red pepper flakes
- 1 ½ lbs chicken breast cut into bite-size pieces
- 10 to 20 drops orange essential oil
- 1/32 tsp powdered stevia (this is optional: Add more if extra sweetness is desired)
- 2 tbsp arrowroot powder (omit for keto diet)
- 2 tbsp sesame seeds

Directions:

1. Use the stainless-steel insert from your instant pot and combine the avocado/coconut oil, coconut aminos, tomato paste, honey, garlic, ginger, bone broth, pepper, and pepper flakes. Whisk these ingredients together.

2. Cut chicken into bite-size pieces and add to the sauce mix.

3. Place the lid on the instant pot and make sure the seal is in place. Close the vent.

4. Press the *manual* or *pressure cook* button and adjust the time to 10 minutes.

5. When you hear the pot beep, release the pressure immediately.

6. Press the *sauté* button and let the sauce come to a simmer.

7. Add the orange essential oil and stir. Taste the contents and add more if you desire. At this time, you can also add a bit more stevia should you want the taste to be sweeter.

8. If you want a sticky, thick sauce, add in the arrowroot powder (unless you are following a keto diet, in which case skip this step).

9. For the final step, stir in sesame seeds and you can serve over your choice of zoodles, spaghetti squash, quinoa, or basmati rice (not keto).

Banish the Bugs

No one enjoys the itch of insect bites, and mosquito bites are just the worst! The itching is bad enough, but those pesky mosquitoes can carry diseases like the Zika virus or West Nile virus.

At the same time, it's important to aim for green solutions to problems like these and to reduce and avoid the use of commercial insect repellents that contain harmful chemicals such as DEET.

Essential oils such as lemon, eucalyptus, peppermint, cinnamon, ylang-ylang, and lemongrass have shown effectiveness in treating and preventing those mosquito bites. For protection, you can add your oils to a carrier oil called neem oil and rub that into your skin.

Practice safety and avoid spraying these too close to your eyes. If you spray a mist to walk through, make sure that you close your mouth and eyes to avoid breathing in the mist.

Homemade Bug Spray

<u>*Ingredients:*</u>

- 10 drops lemon essential oil
- 10 drops lavender essential oil
- 10 drops eucalyptus essential oil
- 15 drops peppermint essential oil
- 20 drops of citronella essential oil
- ½ cups water or neem oil

- 1 4 ounce glass spray bottle

Directions:

1. Add all your essential oils into the glass spray bottle.

2. Fill the rest of the bottle with water or neem oil.

3. Shake to blend. You should shake well before each use.

Homemade Bug Spray #2

- ½ cup distilled water
- 1 tbsp avocado oil
- ½ tbsp witch hazel
- 10 drops citronella essential oil
- 7 to 10 drops lemon essential oil
- 7 to 10 drops orange essential oil
- 10 drops rosemary essential oil
- 12 to 16 ounce amber glass bottle fitted with a sprayer lid

Directions:

1. Always use warm water and a gentle soap to clean your bottle and sprayer in between batches. First, run the soapy water through the sprayer, then again with plain water to rinse it thoroughly.

2. Once your bottle is dry you are ready to begin. Start by pouring in the distilled water. You may want to use a funnel to add some of these ingredients.

3. Add the avocado oil and the witch hazel. Swirl the ingredients together for a few seconds. Set the bottle down and allow the contents to settle.

4. Carefully add the indicated drops above of each essential oil. The order is not important. Shake gently.

5. Your spray is ready to use. Keep your bug spray and your ingredients in a cool, dark place.

6. Make sure to use up this mixture within 6 months so the ingredients remain fresh.

You can trade or add the following essential oils to the mixture if you wish. It's your blend and you can personalize it any way you want to.

- 4 drops geranium essential oil
- 4 drops lemongrass essential oil
- 8 drops eucalyptus essential oil
- 5 drops peppermint essential oil
- 3 drops thyme essential oil
- 6 drops cedar essential oil
- 3 drops clove essential oil

Bed Bug Peppermint Spray

If you do a lot of traveling, you might worry about bringing extra friends home with you. In 2019, researchers performed a study using geraniol, cedar oil, and sod sodium lauryl sulfate which killed over 90% of bed bugs in addition to an 87% mortality rate for their eggs. Below, find a basic essential oil recipe for at-home use.

Ingredients:

- 10 drops peppermint essential oil
- 10 drops clove essential oil
- 3 drops witch hazel
- 100 milliliters (a little more than ⅓ cup) rubbing alcohol. The higher the concentration the better. Aim for a 90% solution.

Directions:

1. Shake all the ingredients together in a glass spray bottle and spray directly on the bed, any bedding, and the surrounding area. Make sure you avoid using the spray near any open flames, electrical sockets, or extension cords.

Again, you can customize your blend any way you like and add or substitute any of the following to the mixture.

- 10 drops lavender essential oil
- 10 drops rosemary essential oil
- 19 drops eucalyptus essential oil

Chapter 4: Using Essential Oils Safely

In general, essential oils are safe to use, but like anything else there are precautions you should follow while using them, especially if you take any prescription medications or are pregnant. In either of these instances, you should only use essential oils under the care of your physician.

In most cases, you should always use a carrier oil when applying oils directly to your skin (especially on your face). I like to test a small patch of skin just to make sure that I am not going to suffer from an allergic reaction. You should always research any oil that you want to use. For example, the citrus essential oils tend to make the wearer's skin more sensitive to sunlight; if you are planning a day at the beach, you may want to hold off on applying orange to your skin.

If you experience any of these symptoms, then you may be experiencing a negative reaction and should stop using the oil immediately:

- Rashes
- Asthma attacks
- Headaches
- Allergic reactions
- Skin Irritation
- Nausea

If you have any surgery planned for an upcoming date, you should avoid the use of essential oils beforehand. Listed below are a few health conditions for which essential oil usage is not recommended. When in doubt, ask your physician.

- Asthma
- High blood pressure
- Epilepsy
- Eczema
- Psoriasis
- Hay Fever

Be cautious because most essential oils are highly concentrated; if you have residue on your hands from using an essential oil, you should take great care not to touch your eyes or get them too close to your nose as this can result in a burning sensation in your mucous membranes. You might think that anything natural would be risk-free, but remember that even natural remedies have the potential to create health consequences when not used correctly. You should know that the essential oil contained in the bottle you hold is fifty to one hundred times more concentrated than the plant it came from. Do your research, be cautious, and speak to a physician if anything seems off.

Dilution Guidelines

Many essential oil recipes and guidelines call for the essential oils to be diluted with a carrier oil. But what exactly *is* a carrier oil? These oils allow you to use your essential oils safely, and often bring added benefits to your health. When you use a carrier oil it allows you to dilute your essential oils to cover a larger area of your body's surface. Using a carrier oil also reduces the chance of negative skin reactions.

Many carrier oils come loaded with essential fatty acids, anti-inflammatory compounds, skin-healing vitamins, and added antioxidants.

Carrier Oils

There are several carrier oils to choose from. In addition to keeping you safe, they also prevent the evaporation of essential oils. If you have ever applied lavender oil directly to your skin, you may notice that after just a few minutes you can no longer smell the scent. That's because it has already been absorbed; when you use a carrier oil the absorption rate will slow down, allowing for a longer application and a more lasting benefit. Read on to learn more about the best carrier oils available.

Coconut Oil

As a carrier, coconut oil has a low molecular weight which allows the compound to penetrate your skin deeper and over a longer period of time. The saturated fats will help your skin to stay moisturized, and you may even notice a smoother and more even skin tone as a result.

Coconut oil is the perfect carrier oil for someone struggling with skin conditions such as acne, eczema, and cold sores because of the antiseptic and antimicrobial properties inherent within this oil.

In every half teaspoon of coconut oil, you can combine one to three drops of any essential oil that is deemed safe for topical use. Afterwards, rub the mixture into the area you wish to address.

Almond Oil

This is a popular carrier oil because it contains antioxidants and also helps to keep your skin soft. Since almond oil is light, it has the ability to absorb deeply into your skin and when used with essential oils like tea tree or lavender you will experience a gentle cleanse all the way down to your pores and follicles. To use this as a carrier oil, combine one to three drops of any topical-safe essential oil with half a teaspoon of almond oil.

Since almond oil contains emollient properties, you may find that it improves your complexion. *Tip: If you are using a reed diffuser, almond oil is light and easily used with this type of application, thereby spreading the scent of the essential oils.*

Jojoba Oil

This is a popular choice because this oil has no odor, and it helps soothe your skin and unclog your pores and hair follicles. Jojoba oil contains three fatty acids and vitamins E and B, which aid in the treatment of sunburn.

Jojoba oil is not truly an oil but instead a plant wax that is a popular moisturizer, cleanser, balancer, and protector of your skin; it helps prevent razor burn and will add to the overall health of your hair. To use this as a carrier oil, combine one to three drops of any topical-safe essential oil with a half teaspoon of jojoba oil.

Olive Oil

Not just for cooking! Olive oil provides beneficial fatty acids as well as anti-inflammatory and antioxidant compounds. When you consume extra virgin olive oil you boost the benefits to your heart and brain, so why wouldn't you consider using it to hydrate your skin, fight infections, and accelerate wound healing? To use this as a carrier oil, combine one to three drops of any topical-safe essential oil with a half teaspoon of olive oil.

Avocado Oil

Just like olive oil, avocado oil not only benefits your health when consumed but also when applied to your skin. This oil adds moisture for people that struggle with rough, dry skin. If you feel the need to hydrate your hair or improve your skin texture, avocado oil might be a great choice for you to use with your essential oils.

You can even use avocado oil alone by simply applying it with a cotton ball to the dry areas on your face, dry hair, or cracked heels. To use this as a carrier oil, combine one to three drops of any topical-safe essential oil with half a teaspoon of avocado oil.

Argan Oil

Using argan oil is a great choice, especially if you have sensitive skin. This oil contains omega-6 fatty acids, linoleic acid, antioxidants, and vitamins A and E, which makes it popular to include in cosmetic products.

This oil will absorb quickly and won't leave you with the feeling of greasy skin. In addition, argan oil is proven to be a carrier that is effective no matter your skin type. To use this as a carrier oil, combine one to three drops of any topical-safe essential oil with a half teaspoon of argan oil.

Arnica Oil

Arnica oil has a proven track record for addressing skin and body issues and is one of the best choices for an essential oil carrier. Because arnica contains helenalin, it is a powerful anti-inflammatory compound and also provides thymol and several fatty acids which will activate antibacterial activity.

Alone, arnica oil is best known as a product that reduces inflammation and muscle pain. As a carrier oil and when paired with lavender and peppermint, you can apply this combination to heal and diminish bruising.

When you read the ingredient label for arnica products, you will notice that it also contains a separate base oil such as olive oil or almond oil. This is significant because arnica is not meant to be used on the skin when it's not diluted. You should also know that arnica oil is not to be meant to be applied to open wounds or cuts. Arnica should also be avoided by women that are breastfeeding or pregnant.

Rosehip Oil

This is another oil that contains essential fatty acids that promote cellular and tissue regeneration. Rosehip has anti-aging properties and is also known to be high in vitamin C. It provides many skin benefits including improving age spots caused by sun damage, and the oil also fights skin infections.

Because rosehip oil is a dry oil, it will be absorbed into your skin quickly but won't leave you with an oily residue, and it works best for people with normal to dry skin. Rosehip oil can also be used alone, in addition to as an essential oil carrier.

Broccoli Seed Oil

This oil is produced by cold-pressing the small seeds of broccoli sprouts. This oil contains high levels of omega 3, 6, and 9 fatty acids.

When using broccoli seed oil, you will probably experience added healing and a reduction in dryness in regard to your hair. This oil works as an excellent moisturizer.

Flaxseed Oil

You are probably used to seeing this oil in your recipes for salads and smoothies, but it also makes a beneficial carrier oil for your essential oils. Flaxseed oil is used in Ayurvedic medicine to balance a person's skin pH levels to promote healing and the removal of skin blemishes.

Flaxseed oil is gentle and a perfect carrier to use when you have sensitive skin. The omega-3 fatty acids and alpha-linoleic acids (ALAs) reduce inflammation and enhance the overall health of your skin and hair.

Grapefruit Seed Extract

You have probably noticed this in the ingredients label of your shower gel, toothpaste, or mouthwash thanks to this carrier's ability to fight bacterial, fungal, and viral infections. In your household you can add this extract to your swimming pool, laundry, or humidifier to reduce the impact of unnecessary harmful chemicals.

Unlike many of the other carriers listed here, you should use equal parts grapefruit seed extract and essential oil. The only way to dilute the combination further is to add another odorless carrier oil to your mixture.

Magnesium Oil

This is another product on my list that is *called* an oil, but isn't really a true oil. Magnesium oil is a mixture of magnesium chloride flakes and water. When combined, this has the same texture as an oil, which is why it can be used as a carrier oil. It works well for people with oily skin because of its ability to break the bond between fats and oils, preventing the formation of a greasy appearance.

When used topically it has been known to improve fibromyalgia symptoms and skin irritations such as rosacea and acne. If you want to use a spray after your shower, combine this and some lavender together and use it after showering.

Neem Oil

This product is found in many natural skin and beauty products because of its high levels of antioxidants. Neem oil has high levels of fatty acids and vitamin E, so it helps relieve dry or damaged skin and is quickly absorbed leaving you feeling grease-free.

Besides its ability to rejuvenate skin cells, neem oil sets itself apart from all the others because it works as a natural insecticide. If you want to fend off flies, mosquitoes, and moths, neem oil can be used alone or mixed with essential oils like eucalyptus or lemon.

If you want to experiment, try combining neem oil with jojoba oil and lavender to produce a wrinkle cream.

Sea Buckthorn Oil

This oil is regularly used to relieve sunburn or speed up healing, but it can also reduce skin irritations such as acne, eczema, or dermatitis. If you have dry or damaged skin in need of repair, this can be an excellent carrier oil to use. Since this oil is filled with healing antioxidants, it will help protect your body from viruses. Like most of the oils on this list, sea buckthorn oil contains essential fatty acids and also offers the user amino acids and vitamins A, C, D, and E.

Evening Primrose Oil

Evening primrose's primary use is to balance hormone levels that can create hot flashes and the inability to stay asleep; it also works as an effective carrier for essential oils.

Because of its ability to be anti-inflammatory, you can easily combine it with tea tree oil to create an antimicrobial combination. With this combination you can boost the overall health of your skin. You can also try some of it in your shampoo to promote hair growth.

Final Thoughts on Carrier Oils

Although the whole point of adding your essential oils to a carrier is to reduce the strength of the oil, you should also do a small skin test patch on the carriers. When experimenting, you want to be sure that you don't have a sensitivity or allergy to the carrier.

If you have inadvertently applied an essential oil without the benefit of a carrier oil and find yourself in some discomfort, go to your kitchen cabinet and grab the olive oil bottle to reduce the strength of the essential oil. If you use water, chances are the burning sensation will either stay the same or increase.

Carrier oils have a shelf life and can turn rancid! If you notice that the scent of your carrier has changed, throw it out and buy a new one. Just like your essential oils, they should be stored in a dark glass jar with a tight-fitting top and kept in your refrigerator or in a cool, dark place.

You can find carrier oils at your local health food store or online.

Chapter 5: Using Essential Oils Safely Around Your Pets

You have done your research and have been diffusing, but one day you notice that Fido or Fluffy isn't acting normally. The reason is that not every essential oil is safe to use around your pets, so if you are an animal lover like myself you will need to go that extra mile to make sure that you are keeping their safety in mind.

There seems to be controversy surrounding the use of essential oils on your pets. A lot of the veterinary community advises to not use essential oils; however, many people including holistic vets use them with great success.

If you are just beginning on your essential oils journey with your pet, I would advise you to begin with lighter applications and then gradually build up amounts based upon how your animal is reacting.

I want to caution you that what works for a dog might not work for a cat or even a horse. Individual animals react differently to oils, and some may be toxic to one animal and not to another. It cannot be stressed enough how important it is to do your homework before using oils on your pets and livestock.

The Raindrop Technique

Horses, chickens, dogs, cats, and many other animals have received regular raindrop therapies. Through the application of oils, the raindrop technique helps to remove toxins from the body. This technique first began in the 1980s thanks to the research of D. Gary Young and a medicine man from the Lakota tribe by the name of Wallace Black Elk.

What is a Raindrop Technique and Why Use it?

The basis upon which the raindrop technique was built was a theory that spinal misalignments and scoliosis are caused by viruses or bacteria that are found lying dormant within the spine. Some horses suffer from a disease called equine protozoal myelitis (EPM). This disease is an infection that operates like a bacteria and can lie dormant in a horse's central nervous system for years until for unknown reasons it will activate and create a bout of illness, with symptoms like hindlimb weakness or muscle atrophy. I mention this because there is a raindrop therapy for horses specifically aimed at relieving EPM.

A raindrop technique will use a specific sequence of essential oils that are antimicrobial in nature to reduce inflammation and attack any lurking viral agents. The basic single oils used for a raindrop are listed below. You should be aware that any raindrop therapy can vary depending upon the animal in question.

- Thyme (Thymus vulgaris)
- Oregano (Origanum compactum)

- Wintergreen/birch (Gaultheria procumberas, Betula alleghaniensis)
- Cypress (Cupressus sempervirens)
- Peppermint (Menta piperita)
- Basil (Ocimum basilicum)
- Marjoram (Origanum majorana)

Each will have a designated number of drops and application directions that will depend upon the recipient. While this technique was originally designed for humans, there are many animal versions that even a beginner will be able to perform with confidence.

When applying the oils to animals each oil will be dropped on the spine area from a distance of about six inches above the subject from head to tail. One large difference between the human and animal techniques is that humans generally have the raindrop applied to their feet. Most smaller animals do not tolerate the application to their paws or pads. The only noted exception to this is when treating horses, which are more accepting when it comes to applying oils to the hoof or leg area.

You will need to read up on the specifics for the species you are treating, but the application of raindrop oils will start at the tail and travel along the spine to the base of the head.

Because animals are often moving targets you should be careful when approaching the area around the base of the neck. Should they look up to see what you are doing, you could mistakenly drop oil near an eye or nose. Take care to avoid these sensitive areas.

Stroking in the Oils

After the oil is applied up the back, you will need to stroke it into the back of the animal. There are varying techniques to use, and there is not one that is better than the others. There are no rules to follow, just find a technique that works for both you and your animal. Depending upon the animal's coat, you may need to alter your technique.

Generally speaking, the stroking of each individual oil application is repeated three times. You can also use a carrier oil for your animals, and I recommend a V-6 enhanced vegetable oil complex. It is a thinner oil that not only absorbs well but also works well with fur and feathers. If you cannot locate this carrier, you can use coconut oil or olive oil instead.

Raindrop Example: Cat

I am including an example of a raindrop for one species. According to Doctor of Veterinary Medicine Melissa Shelton (a specialist in Veterinary Aromatic Medicine), the following technique was created by Leigh Foster, a woman who runs a large cat rescue and has used essential oils on many rescue cats. Despite essential oils often being controversial when used with animals, this technique has been found to have some amazing results for both veterinarians and owners alike.

Kitty Raindrop:
<u>Oils:</u>

- Oregano

- Thyme
- Basil
- Cypress
- Wintergreen
- Marjoram
- Peppermint

Application:

1. Add 4 drops of each of the above oils to a 1 ounce glass bottle, then add V-6 or another appropriate carrier to fill the remainder of the bottle.

2. Mix the contents by gently rocking the bottle back and forth.

3. Apply approximately 6 drops of the solution up the spine of the cat from tail to head.

4. Gently stroke the essential oil solution up the back of the cat working from the tail to the head. Surprisingly, most cats will not object to this step; however, should they, you can pet your cat normally or leave out the strokes completely.

5. You can repeat this up to three times during one session.

Conclusion

Throughout these pages you have been provided with some of the interesting histories regarding the discovery of essential oils through their early uses and how it was often the initial go-to for medicines and healthcare professionals.

I have listed many of the maladies that essential oils are used to treat, covering physical, mental, and emotional well-being. The scent of these oils affects our limbic system, which is connected to parts of our brain that can influence our body and how we think.

Chapter one provided you with a list of essential oils that are considered some of the most commonly used foundation oils and are a perfect start to any practice. You do not need to have all the oils and can get started with just a basic five or so to begin your journey. Everyone has different needs which require different oils. Remember that if there is one oil you must have, start with lavender. It has many benefits and is one of the most versatile oils.

In regard to the oils, we have discussed how to pick quality oils that are beneficial as opposed to lesser quality oils that can be filled with harmful additives which may end up harming you instead of helping you. In addition to this, you have been given tips on how to tell a real oil from a fake one.

The art of using essential oils is commonly referred to as aromatherapy, and while describing all the benefits of aromatherapy I have given you a list of applications that you can use to experience the holistic health benefits for yourself. While reading through the various ways to experience aromatherapy, I am sure that you will come up with a favorite or three! Diffusing is the most popular manner of oil utilization, but if you need to carry something with you at work or while you are on the go, an aromatic spritzer or an aromatherapy inhaler might make it easier to access your favorite oils.

If you have specific symptoms you are trying to manage, an aromatherapist may also be able to lend a hand and make some suggestions to help you manage your approach.

You can always treat yourself right in your own home. Take a soothing bath filled with your homemade blends of bath salts to provide a calming experience. You can follow it up with your homemade lotions that compliment your bath salts. If you are still in need of some spa time, break out that facial steamer, add some essential oils, and treat your skin to a session that will cleanse your pores and revitalize your skin. Doing all this before bedtime will make your slumber long and uninterrupted.

There are thousands of ways to use essential oils creatively, and I have provided a list for you along with some of my favorite recipes to enjoy.

Like any medicine or application, there are some safety precautions that you should take when using essential oils. A little goes a very long way, and many make the mistake of indulging in the use of them without first checking the basic safety guidelines. Many of the oils when used at full strength can cause uncomfortable sensations, which is why it is important to know about carriers and doing small patch testing.

Finally, if you have pets in your household, take special precautions when choosing and using essential oils. I cannot stress enough how important it is to do your homework when it comes to using essential oils around animals. Not every essential oil is safe for pets, and some can be safe for your dog but toxic for your cat.

However, your pets and livestock can also enjoy benefits from essential oils. Every time my dog is stressed, I reach for the lavender and apply just a drop to his paw pads to help calm him.

Enjoy your journey into the use and practice of essential oils; in addition to bringing about fantastic scents and calming aromas, they can bring great relief and make you feel better physically, mentally, spiritually, and emotionally.

www.ingramcontent.com/pod-product-compliance
Lightning Source LLC
LaVergne TN
LVHW011738060526
838200LV00051B/3237